Beyond the Letters

Winning the Dyslexia Battle

By Chris Roberts

TABLE OF CONTENTS

INTRODUCTION

Accepting the Journey
Hello and welcome to "Beyond the Letters: Winning the Dyslexia Battle". We set out on a path of comprehension, resiliency, and victory over the difficulties presented by dyslexia on these pages. This introduction acts as our road map, helping you navigate the dyslexic terrain, busting misconceptions along the way, and showing you how to overcome dyslexia rather than simply cope with it.

Getting Around the Terrain
A Definition of Dyslexia

Dyslexia, which is often misinterpreted, involves more than just trouble with writing and reading. It's a distinct brain characteristic that affects how people interpret information. In these first chapters, we dissect dyslexia to reveal its actual nature, delving beyond popular descriptions to understand its subtleties.

Effect on Persons

Dyslexia has a variety of effects on people's lives, including both adults and children. Destroying stereotypes and promoting an inclusive society need an understanding of its effects. This chapter explores the daily lives of people who have dyslexia, providing insight into the difficulties they encounter as well as the advantages they possess.

The Empowering Power of Knowledge

Our goal as we delve into the nuances of dyslexia is to empower as much as to educate. To break down the obstacles that misunderstandings and biases create, knowledge is essential. With the proper knowledge, you, the reader, will be more capable of navigating the path that lies ahead, whether it is for a loved one, yourself, or just to promote understanding in your community.

Seeing Past Restraints

A Change in Paradigm

This book is a call to action to change the way we think about dyslexia—from seeing it as a disability to seeing it as a distinct way of seeing the world. This paradigm shift is expanded upon in each chapter, leading to a celebration of the contributions that people with dyslexia make to society.

CHAPTER 1: Myths and Facts about Dyslexia

Deconstructing the Tapestry
In the first chapter of "Beyond the Letters," we set out on a deep examination to debunk the misconceptions surrounding dyslexia and to shed light on the information that forms the basis of our groundbreaking investigation. It's time to reassemble the complex puzzle that has for far too long obscured dyslexia.

The Mythological Veil Dispelling Myths
Myths surrounding dyslexia, which is often misinterpreted, have been reinforced by false information and ignorance. We methodically demolish these myths in this chapter, exposing the origins of widely accepted ideas and illuminating the reality behind the illness. We enable ourselves to confront dyslexia with never-before-seen clarity and purpose by distinguishing reality from myth.

First misconception: Dyslexia only affects reading and writing.
Factual statement: Dyslexia is a complex neurological disorder that extends beyond reading. Even though dyslexia may cause difficulties with reading and writing, it also affects other areas of cognitive functioning including memory, organizing abilities, and even creative thought.

Second misconception: People with dyslexia are not intellectual.
Fact: Dyslexia does not impair intelligence. In actuality, a large number of dyslexic people have extraordinary abilities in domains like creativity, spatial thinking, and problem-solving. We explore the studies and provide anecdotes that highlight the variety of talents possessed by dyslexic brains.

Dyslexia's Actualities Outside of Reading and Writing
One common misconception is that dyslexia only affects a person's ability to read and write. This chapter expands on that viewpoint by exploring the complexity of dyslexia. We challenge the constrictive myths that have limited our knowledge by revealing the many effects dyslexia has on people, ranging from cognitive processing to creativity.

The Cognitive Spectrum: Dyslexia has a distinct impact on cognitive functions. We examine how spatial thinking, creativity, and problem-solving may be strong points for dyslexic people, providing a comprehensive understanding of their cognitive abilities.

Unleashed Creativity: Despite popular assumptions, dyslexia often coexists with increased creativity. We debunk the myth that dyslexia is just a restricting disease by examining how the distinctive thought processes of dyslexic individuals foster creativity and creative expression.

An Exploration of Misunderstood Historical Viewpoints

Following the Origins

We take a historical tour to understand the history of attitudes and ideas around dyslexia and to properly comprehend the current. We may obtain insight into the roots of popular myths and provide the foundation for a more informed discourse by comprehending the historical backdrop.

Ancient Perceptions: We can find early records of people with dyslexia dating back to ancient civilizations. Even if the language changed, the identification of distinct cognitive processes shows how dyslexia has persisted throughout history.

Middle Ages and Later: Dyslexia was often misconstrued as a sign of intellectual weakness or sloth throughout the Middle Ages. We examine how cultural beliefs shaped how people with dyslexia were treated, setting the stage for centuries of miscommunication.

Development of Modern Understanding: During the 19th and 20th centuries, attitudes changed as early psychologists started to identify dyslexia as a separate disorder. We explore the important roles and turning points that cleared the path for a more complex comprehension.

Forming the Story
Culture, Media, and Dyslexia: The media is crucial in influencing how society views things. This section analyzes and assesses the influence and authenticity of popular cultural depictions of dyslexia. By addressing preconceptions head-on, we create the foundation for a conversation that is more thoughtful and kind.

Portrayals in Literature and Film: We examine how dyslexia is portrayed in different media and consider how this affects public opinion. We address prejudices that lead to misperception as well as positive depictions that foster understanding.

The Stigma Language: Expressions count. We examine the vocabulary that is used in public discourse around dyslexia, calling attention to stigmatizing phrases and promoting a language change that is more empowering and kind.

An Appeal for Knowledge
Fighting for the Truth: Equipped with this newfound understanding, we close this chapter determined to debunk misconceptions about dyslexia. It's a call to action to replace ignorance with knowledge and create an atmosphere that supports the success of people with dyslexia.

Educational Initiatives: We discuss current initiatives to provide correct information on dyslexia in the curriculum for schools. By promoting truth in education, we open the door for a future generation that recognizes and values neurodiversity.

Community Involvement: Raising consciousness goes beyond the classroom. We examine grassroots groups and neighborhood projects that aim to debunk misconceptions about dyslexia to build a culture that is more accepting and encouraging

CHAPTER 2: Symptoms of Dyslexia in Adults and Children

Getting Around the Signs
In "Beyond the Letters," chapter two, we go on a trip that examines dyslexia symptoms in great detail. This chapter emphasizes the value of early detection and intervention and acts as a crucial reference for identifying important signs in both adults and children.

Early Symptoms in Kids
It's essential to comprehend the signs of dyslexia in kids to encourage early detection and provide appropriate assistance. This section explores the non-obvious and obvious symptoms that may point to dyslexia in young children.

Delayed Speech Development: A delay in speech development is a common early sign. We examine how articulation and language acquisition issues may serve as early indicators of dyslexia, emphasizing the need for vigilant parenting and expert assessment.

Difficulties with Phonological Awareness: The ability to recognize sounds in words is a prerequisite for reading. We examine in detail how children with dyslexia may struggle with sound recognition and manipulation, which may hinder their comprehension of written language.

Difficulties with Visual and Auditory Processing: Dyslexia often causes problems with the processing of both visual and auditory information. We look at how these issues might show up in a child's day-to-day functioning and how it affects their comprehension and response to spoken and written language.

Executive Functioning Difficulties: Dyslexia may affect executive functions such as planning, organizing, and working memory in addition to language-specific issues. We look at how these difficulties could impact a child's everyday activities and academic achievement.

Acknowledging Adult Difficulties Lifelong Views
Dyslexia doesn't go away in childhood: it follows a person for the rest of their life. This section explores the signs and difficulties that individuals with dyslexia encounter, highlighting the need for ongoing education and assistance.

Reading and Workplace Issues: Dyslexia may cause problems in a variety of spheres of everyday life as an adult, particularly in the workplace. We examine the potential effects on a person's career of difficulties in reading work papers, comprehending directions, and writing down ideas.

Adults with dyslexia often come up with compensating techniques to get around obstacles. We explore the creative ways people adjust, demonstrating resiliency and flexibility in the face of diversity in lifelong learning.

Emotional and Psychological Aspects: Self-worth and general well-being may be impacted by dyslexia. We examine the psychological and emotional aspects of having dyslexia, emphasizing the value of mental health resources and cultivating a positive self-concept.

A Way to Comprehend Early Intervention and Assistance, Strengthening Families and Teachers
Early dyslexia recognition facilitates successful therapy. This section emphasizes cooperative efforts between families, educators, and experts as it examines different tactics and approaches that might benefit children with dyslexia in school settings.

Educational adjustments: To foster an inclusive learning environment, we examine the significance of putting adjustments into place in schools. We look at resources that give dyslexic pupils more control, such as assistive technology and individualized lesson plans.

Parental Guidance: Parents are essential in identifying and helping their dyslexic children. We provide advice on how to promote candid communication, comprehend the nature of education, and speak out in support of their child's needs.

Community Resources: Emphasizing resources outside of the classroom, we investigate organizations and community-based support systems devoted to raising awareness of dyslexia. Making these materials available to families promotes a feeling of belonging and mutual understanding.

Systems of Adult Support
Getting Around Workplaces and More: The significance of support networks for adults with dyslexia is covered in this section. We look at ways to develop success and resilience in several facets of adult life, such as self-advocacy and employment adjustments.

Workplace Inclusivity: We talk about how organizations may foster inclusive environments that use the abilities of their dyslexic staff members. We emphasize methods that are advantageous to both people and companies, ranging from assistive technology to flexible work arrangements.

Developing Personal Tactics: People with dyslexia often come up with original success tactics. We share first-hand accounts and life lessons to encourage those who are struggling to deal with dyslexia as adults.

From Acknowledgment to Promotion
As this chapter draws to an end, it is clear that comprehending the symptoms of dyslexia involves more than simply identification—rather, it involves a continuum that extends from advocacy to recognition. By recognizing the symptoms in both kids and adults, we help create a culture where people with dyslexia are actively supported and encouraged, despite their unique neurodevelopmental characteristics.

CHAPTER 3: The Causes and Types of Dyslexia

The Neurological Tapestry

In "Beyond the Letters," chapter three, we take a deep dive into the causes and subtleties of dyslexia, revealing the intricate neural fabric that forms this particular neurodevelopmental disorder.

Comprehending Neurological Elements

The Intricate Origins: The complex neurological roots of dyslexia go deep into the body. This section delves into a thorough analysis of the many elements that lead to the development of dyslexia, providing a sophisticated knowledge of the complex interactions between brain shape, genetics, and cognitive processes.

Genetic Influences: A thorough investigation of the genetic foundations of dyslexia is the first step in the quest. We make our way across the complex genetic terrain, pinpointing certain genes linked to differences in the way the brain develops language and reading abilities. We can learn a great deal about the hereditary components of dyslexia and how genetic predispositions affect people's experiences and family patterns.

Brain Structure and Function: We continue our neuroscientific investigation by delving into state-of-the-art brain imaging research. These investigations provide a clearer knowledge of how these neurological variants affect language processing by revealing the structural and functional abnormalities in the brains of people with dyslexia. Cortical areas, brain pathways, and connection patterns are all covered in the debate, offering a wealth of information about the neuroscience of dyslexia.

Subtypes and Differences

Far from being a single, universal disorder, dyslexia may take many different shapes and intensities. This section delves into a thorough examination of the many dyslexia subtypes and variants, illuminating the distinctive traits that distinguish each subtype.

Phonological Dyslexia: We explore the complex realm of phonological dyslexia, a subtype marked by difficulties understanding spoken language sounds. The study covers the brain's phonological processing pathways, revealing how problems with phoneme recognition and manipulation appear and affect the comprehension of written words.

Surface Dyslexia: As we examine surface dyslexia, visual word recognition takes center stage. Problems with irregular words—words that don't follow standard phonetic patterns—are part of this group. The conversation delves into the nuances of visual processing, providing insight into how people with surface dyslexia deal with the complexity of written language.

Fast Naming Deficit: An in-depth analysis of fast naming deficits sheds light on the difficulties that members of this subtype encounter. The conversation also covers the cognitive processes included in swiftly identifying letters, colors, or recognizable things, and how impairments in these areas lead to difficulties with reading comprehension and fluency.

Double-Deficit Dyslexia: This subtype of dyslexia involves problems with both phonological processing and quick naming. We explore the many obstacles associated with double-deficit dyslexia. The investigation takes into account how these deficiencies are reinforced and highlights the need for focused treatments that cover a variety of reading-related topics.

Success is Nurtured by Environmental and Educational Factors

Apart from the neurological aspects, the experiences of persons with dyslexia are significantly shaped by environmental and educational variables. This section offers a thorough examination of how focused interventions and a supportive atmosphere may foster success.

Early Literacy Experiences: We explore the fundamental effects that early literacy experiences have on those who are dyslexic. The investigation covers how rich literacy settings may encourage a love of language and reading in children from a young age. The significance of establishing a loving early learning environment is emphasized in the strategies for parents, caregivers, and educators that are covered.

Educational Interventions: The importance of individualized approaches in the classroom is highlighted by a thorough analysis of evidence-based interventions and instructional strategies. The usefulness of multimodal approaches, organized literacy programs, and assistive technology in meeting the various demands of dyslexic people is covered in the debate. We examine how educational interventions are changing while taking research and practice into account.

Accepting Neurodiversity: In this part, we examine the idea of accepting neurodiversity in educational contexts and propose a paradigm change. The conversation questions deficit-focused methods and promotes appreciating and celebrating dyslexic people's talents. A neurodiverse perspective's transformational ability is emphasized via the specific strategies for establishing inclusive and empowered learning settings.

Customizing Interventions and Support
A strong focus is made on the value of individualized assistance and interventions as this chapter comes to a close. A deeper insight that goes beyond generalizations is established by investigating causes and subtypes. We open the door for focused strategies that value variety and develop each person's potential by appreciating and appreciating the distinctive abilities of every person on the dyslexia spectrum.

CHAPTER 4: Diagnosis and Evaluation of Dyslexia

Early Warning Signs and Screening Identifying Concerns

Parents and teachers are essential in spotting any dyslexia symptoms in kids. Early detection depends on open dialogue and teamwork.

Educator and Parental Observations: Create a supportive atmosphere where early indications of dyslexia may be recognized and swiftly treated by encouraging educators and parents to actively observe and record any symptoms.

Formal and Informal Screening Measures: To determine a child's dyslexia risk, use a variety of screening measures such as teacher observations and standardized examinations. These resources provide insightful information on a child's learning profile.

All-inclusive Evaluation

Exposing the Intricacy

To comprehend the complexity of dyslexia and customize therapies to meet the requirements of each person, a thorough examination is necessary.

Psychoeducational Evaluation: To evaluate social-emotional aspects, academic performance, and cognitive ability, conduct psychoeducational examinations. Personalized therapies are built on this comprehensive approach.

Utilize neuropsychological testing to identify certain cognitive processes—such as memory, attention, and executive functions—that are associated with dyslexia. These evaluations provide a detailed picture of each person's learning profile.

Use dynamic assessment techniques that provide real-time insights into learning processes by responding to each person's answer. Personalized interventions are aided by these evaluations.

Interdisciplinary cooperation bridging viewpoints
Working across disciplines is essential to developing a thorough knowledge of dyslexia. Collaboration between educators, psychologists, speech-language pathologists, and other experts is recommended.

Collaborate as a team in educational environments to ensure that instructors, special educators, and support workers work well together. This collaboration creates a cohesive support approach by incorporating evaluations into customized lesson plans.

Gain insights from a variety of disciplines by using the work of occupational therapists and speech-language pathologists, among others. Working together expands the assessment's focus by taking into account a variety of dyslexia-influencing elements.

Parental Involvement: Stress the importance of parents' participation in the evaluation process. Promote parental involvement, advocacy, and teamwork with experts to deepen the understanding of each child's distinct requirements.

From Evaluation to Involvement

Creating Customized Support Programs
Customized assistance plans are developed based on insights gained from the diagnostic process, enabling dyslexic persons to achieve both personal and academic success.

Individualized Education Plans (IEPs): Create and carry out IEPs following the results of assessments. These plans act as guides for teachers, providing particular interventions and modifications to meet individual requirements.

Response to Intervention (RTI): Put the Response to Intervention (RTI) framework into practice, emphasizing early intervention techniques to stop academic difficulties from becoming worse. The requirements of every student are met thanks to this tiered assistance system.

Technological Interventions: Examine how assistive technology and specialized software may be used to serve dyslexic people. These resources improve educational opportunities and support students' academic progress.

CHAPTER 5: Treatment and Intervention Options for Dyslexia

Getting Around the Support Environment

In the fifth chapter of "Beyond the Letters," we examine the wide range of dyslexia intervention and treatment methods. This chapter provides a thorough overview, illuminating evidence-based tactics, assistive technology, and focused methods that help people with dyslexia succeed in school.

Interventions Based on Phonics

Establishing Bases
The cornerstone of dyslexia assistance is phonics-based therapies, which emphasize the underlying abilities required for reading.

Explore evidence-based programs for organized literacy that teach word recognition, decoding, and phonics methodically. These courses provide a methodical approach while meeting each student's unique requirements.

Multimodal Approaches: Stress the value of using multimodal approaches that include the visual, aural, and kinesthetic senses. These experiential methods improve learning by engaging the senses in different ways.

Assistive Technology

Enhancing Education
The use of assistive technology is crucial in providing tools that enable academic performance and learning for those with dyslexia.

Text-to-Speech Software: Examine the advantages of this technology that enables people to hear written text. This technology promotes various learning styles and aids with understanding.

Applications for Speech-to-Text: Explore applications that allow users to dictate their ideas. This helps overcome obstacles in textual communication.

Customizable Fonts and Backgrounds: Stress the significance of having editable fonts and color backdrops for digital content. For those with dyslexia, these elements improve reading and lessen visual stress.

Modifications and Accommodations for Reading

Customizing the Educational Setting
To meet the specific requirements of people with dyslexia, the learning environment must include accommodations and adjustments.

Longer Time Allotted for Tasks and Assessments: Promote longer time limits for tasks and evaluations. With this concession, people with dyslexia may demonstrate their comprehension without any time limits.

Use of Audiobooks: Promote the use of audiobooks as a substitute for printed books. Auditory help is provided via audiobooks, which facilitate effective material access for those with dyslexia.

Examine the advantages that come with using graphic organizers and visual aids. By arranging information, these tools promote understanding and help with memory retention.

Customizing Educational Experiences using Individualized Educational Plans (IEPs)
Developing and implementing Individualized Education Plans (IEPs) is essential to modifying the educational experience for dyslexic students.

Targeted Reading Interventions: Create focused reading programs within the IEP framework. These therapies target certain needs, including fluency in reading or decoding abilities.

Emphasize the need for continuous progress monitoring and adjustments. Frequent evaluations enable teachers to modify intervention tactics based on data, guaranteeing ongoing improvement.

Collaboration Amongst Specialists and Teachers: Encourage cooperation amongst specialists, general educators, and special educators. This multidisciplinary approach guarantees a thorough comprehension of the learner's requirements and efficiently synchronizes treatments.

Constructing a Helpful Ecosystem

Advocacy and Community Resources
As we get to the close of this chapter, our attention turns to creating a healthy ecology outside of the classroom.

Emphasize the importance of community-based support networks, such as parent organizations and advocacy groups for dyslexia. These networks provide a forum for exchanging knowledge, materials, and group advocacy.

Promoting continuous professional development for educators is something you should do. Providing educators with the skills and resources they need to assist students with dyslexia promotes an inclusive classroom.

Encouraging Dyslexia Awareness: Underline how crucial it is to encourage dyslexia awareness in institutions and communities. Raising awareness promotes an inclusive society by lowering stigma and creating better understanding and acceptance.

CHAPTER 6: Strategies and Tools to Overcome Dyslexia

Encouraging People on Their Path

In the sixth chapter of "Beyond the Letters," we explore a variety of methods and resources intended to assist people in conquering the difficulties related to dyslexia. This chapter functions as a helpful manual, providing a toolkit of practical strategies that promote self-assurance, resiliency, and achievement.

Developing Cognitive Capabilities

A key component of recovering dyslexia is developing cognitive skills, which focuses on improving certain cognitive functions that are essential for reading and comprehension.

Memory Enhancement Strategies: Examine strategies for improving memory that support knowledge retention. Repetition, imagery, and mnemonic devices all help to create a strong basis for remembering.

Exercises for Auditory Processing: Practice processing and interpreting spoken language by participating in exercises for auditory processing. Improved comprehension and phonological awareness are two benefits of these workouts.

Executive Function Techniques: Put techniques in place to help with time management, planning, and organizing. These resources enable people to successfully manage everyday and academic responsibilities.

Supportive Techniques for Reading

For people with dyslexia, reading assistive methods are essential in increasing their accessibility to written content.

Color Overlays and Filters: Use color overlays and filters to improve reading comfort and lessen visual strain. Both digital displays and printed documents may be used with these instruments.

instruments for Guided Reading: To improve attention and concentration, use instruments for guided reading such as reading rulers or guides. By minimizing visual distractions, these technologies assist readers in staying focused.

Encourage text annotation and highlighting as useful techniques for improving reading comprehension. These techniques support better comprehension overall, attentional concentration, and identification of important information.

Technology-Oriented Approaches

Technology-based solutions provide creative methods to help dyslexic people in the digital era.

Accept voice recognition software: This technology converts spoken words into text. With the use of this technology, people may express themselves in writing and successfully communicate their ideas.

changeable Fonts and Backgrounds: Use digital devices' changeable fonts and backdrop options to improve reading. Customizing a text's visual elements reduces visual strain and encourages a more pleasant reading experience.

Applications and Games for Education: Look through applications and games that help strengthen reading abilities. These interactive resources provide chances for ongoing skill improvement and make learning interesting.

Self-Support and Mentality

Developing a positive outlook and strengthening self-advocacy abilities are essential components of the dyslexia recovery process.

Attend self-advocacy seminars to acquire the skills people need to express their demands and ask for the adjustments they need. Giving people the freedom to express themselves promotes independence.

Reduce Stress and Practice Mindfulness: Include stress-reduction methods and mindfulness exercises in everyday activities. These techniques support anxiety management, improve concentration, and provide a supportive learning atmosphere.

Celebrating Strengths and Achievements: Encourage the development of a culture that recognizes the special talents and accomplishments of dyslexic people. Acknowledging successes promotes confidence and a good self-image.

Building a Network of Support
Including the Family and the Community
By the end of the chapter, the emphasis will be on creating a network of support that includes the community, educators, and families.

Family Engagement seminars: Arrange for seminars that provide families with useful tips on how to help dyslexic family members at home. Creating a cooperative relationship between the family and the school improves support in general.

Implement training programs for educators to provide them with the tools they need to help dyslexic pupils. Opportunities for professional development help create a more inclusive learning environment.

Community-Based Initiatives: Promote community-based programs that increase dyslexia awareness. Creating a community that recognizes and values neurodiversity promotes a welcoming and supportive atmosphere.

CHAPTER 7: Success Stories and Role Models for Dyslexic People

Motivating Adventures and Successes

In "Beyond the Letters," chapter seven, we explore real-life success stories and highlight prominent individuals who have not only overcome dyslexia's obstacles but also emerged as powerful role models. This chapter honors the fortitude, tenacity, and remarkable accomplishments of those who overcame dyslexia by using their special talents.

Individual Stories

1. Sir Richard Branson: Sir Richard Branson, a well-known businessman, the man behind the Virgin Group, and a dyslexic illustrates through his experience the power of imagination and perseverance. Even though he had difficulty in school, he went on to create a multinational company empire, demonstrating the entrepreneurial drive that dyslexia is frequently linked to.

2. Steven Spielberg: Known for being one of the most recognizable directors in history, Spielberg has been transparent about his dyslexia. His story serves as a testament to how imagination and a distinct viewpoint can produce unmatched success in the entertainment and artistic sectors.

3. Dr. Temple Grandin: A well-known authority on autism advocacy and animal science, Dr. Temple Grandin is dyslexic as well. Her narrative highlights how accepting neurodiversity may result in ground-breaking accomplishments and significant contributions to academics.

Acknowledging Particular Proficiencies Using Neurodiversity

1. Kamprad Ingvar: Ingvar Kamprad, the creator of IKEA, had dyslexia and had difficulty in school in his early years. His achievement in creating one

of the biggest furniture merchants in the world serves as an example of the connection between dyslexia, entrepreneurship, and creative thinking.

2. Agatha Christie: Dyslexic, the renowned mystery writer Agatha Christie is renowned for her unmatched inventiveness and storytelling. Her writing accomplishments serve as evidence of the influence dyslexic people may have in the creative and literary fields.

3. Sir James Dyson: The businessman and developer of Dyson vacuum cleaners, Sir James Dyson, credits his dyslexia for inspiring his creative thinking. His narrative demonstrates how dyslexic people may succeed in engineering and progress technology.

Various Fields' Role Models

1. Dr. Sally Shaywitz: Leading dyslexia researcher Dr. Sally Shaywitz has pushed for the rights of dyslexic people in addition to making a substantial contribution to our knowledge of the condition. Her work has had a long-lasting influence on educational interventions and policy.

2. Whoopi Goldberg: The well-known comedian, actress, and TV personality has disclosed that she has dyslexia. Her career path in entertainment motivates budding artists by showcasing the range of skills within the dyslexic community.

3. Richard Rogers: The renowned, dyslexic architect Richard Rogers is the creator of famous structures like the Pompidou Center in Paris. His contributions to architecture show how dyslexic people may succeed in creative and design-oriented industries.

Putting together a tapestry of Support Systems and Inspirational Resources provides information about services and support networks that people with dyslexia may use for community, inspiration, and direction in addition to these experiences.

1. Drs. Brock and Fernette Eide's book The Dyslexic Advantage: This book examines the special abilities connected to dyslexia and offers advice on how people may make the most of these abilities to succeed.

2. The International Dyslexia Association (IDA) is a respectable group that provides advocacy, information, and support to people with dyslexia and their families.

3. Understood.org: An online resource that offers parents, educators, and people with learning and attention problems tools, community support, and professional assistance.

CHAPTER 8: Resources and Support for Dyslexic People and their Families

Creating a Helpful Network

In "Beyond the Letters," chapter eight, we concentrate on offering an all-inclusive reference to services and support networks designed especially for dyslexics and their families. The goal of this chapter is to provide readers with useful knowledge, resources, and links to help them deal with the difficulties brought on by dyslexia.

Resources for Education Promoting Learning

1. Learning Ally: To help people with dyslexia succeed academically, this charity provides audiobooks and other helpful tools.

2. Bookshare: An easily navigable virtual library that offers a significant selection of electronic books to people with dyslexia and other reading difficulties.

3. International Dyslexia Association (IDA): To advance dyslexia awareness and efficient teaching techniques, IDA provides a plethora of materials, such as webinars, events, and publications.

Utilizing Assistive Technology to Increase Accessibility

1. Ghotit Author and Reader: This assistive technology provides sophisticated grammar and spell checking, which benefits people with dyslexia.

2. Kurzweil 3000: An all-inclusive platform for assistive technology that offers text-to-speech, highlighting, and other capabilities to help with understanding and reading.

3. Dragon NaturallySpeaking: This voice recognition software enables people to dictate text, making it easier for dyslexics to express themselves in writing.

Assistance Institutions Linking Communities
First, the National Center for Learning Impairments (NCLD) offers information, advocacy, and support to people with learning impairments, including dyslexia.

2. Decoding Dyslexia is a grassroots movement that promotes evidence-based methods, policy, and understanding of dyslexia. Local help is provided by state chapters.

3. Yale Center for Dyslexia & Creativity: This center provides tools, research updates, and educational outreach to bridge the gap between research and practice.

Parental Assistance Leading Families
1. Understood.org: An extensive site that provides parents of kids with learning and attention problems with knowledge, assistance, and useful guidance.

2. Parent Training and Information Centers (PTIs): These centers help parents of children with disabilities by giving them information and assistance as well as advice on how to work through the educational system.

3. Bright Solutions for Dyslexia: Started by Susan Barton, this group provides teachers and parents with tools and training to help them assist students with dyslexia.

Legal Support and Advocacy to Uphold Rights
1. Council for Exceptional Children (CEC): To guarantee that people with exceptionalities, such as dyslexia, have access to high-quality education, CEC offers resources and advocacy.

2. Disability Rights Education & Defense Fund (DREDF): This group provides materials and legal advocacy to advance the civil and human rights of those with disabilities.

3. Wrightslaw: An invaluable site that offers parents, educators, and activists information on advocacy and special education law.

Financial Support and Scholarships

1. Allegra and Anne Ford Scholarships Thomas: These scholarships, which are provided by the National Center for Learning Disabilities, assist those who struggle with dyslexia and other learning and attention disorders.

2. The American Learning Disabilities Association (LDA) Scholarships: Students with learning difficulties who choose to pursue higher education might get financial aid from LDA.

3. The Dyslexia Foundation: This organization recognizes the potential of dyslexic kids by providing scholarships and encouraging their academic endeavors.

Virtual Communities Connecting People Online

1. Reddit's Dyslexia Support Forum: An online community where people may connect with others going through similar struggles, exchange stories, and ask for guidance.

2. DyslexiaHelp at the University of Michigan: An online resource offering guidance, tactics, and assistance to parents, teachers, and students with dyslexia.

3. Intelligent Children with Learning Challenges Online Community: This is a virtual community that provides parents of kids with learning challenges, such as dyslexia, with information and support.

Neighborhood-Based Assistance Local Networks

1. Local Decoding Dyslexia Chapters: Decoding Dyslexia chapters may be found in many areas. They plan events, provide support groups, and push for state and local legislative reforms.

2. Parent-Teacher Associations (PTAs): Get involved with your neighborhood PTA to promote dyslexia awareness and push for supportive school policies.

3. Community Libraries: Libraries often provide seminars, activities, and resources to help people and children with dyslexia.

Constructing Future Bridges

The goal of this chapter's conclusion is to provide readers with a wide variety of tools and networks of support, promoting a feeling of empowerment and community. The goal is to point dyslexics and their families in the direction of helpful resources and relationships that will further their journey beyond the letters.

CHAPTER 9: The Future and Hope for Dyslexia

Accepting Development and Opportunities

In "Beyond the Letters," the ninth and last chapter, we examine how dyslexia awareness, education, and assistance are changing. This chapter offers an optimistic outlook for the future, imagining a society in which dyslexia is recognized as a distinctive aspect of human uniqueness rather than as a barrier to achievement.

Research and Understanding Advances Opening Up New Horizons

1. Advances in Neuroscience: Examine current neuroscientific findings that provide insight into the fundamental brain processes linked to dyslexia. These findings assist in a better comprehension of the ailment and guide focused therapies.

2. Genetic Research: Examine current genetic research to find putative genetic markers linked to dyslexia. Personalized therapies based on individual genetic profiles are a promising development in the rapidly developing science of genomics.

Technological and Educational Innovations

1. UDL stands for Universal Design for Learning. Examine the ways that inclusive learning environments that support a range of learning requirements, including dyslexics, are being created by incorporating the concepts of Universal Design for Learning (UDL) into educational practices.

2. Gamification and Interactive Learning: Talk about how educational platforms may include gamification and interactive learning techniques to make learning interesting and cater to the needs of dyslexic students.

Developments in Policy and Advocacy

1. Initiatives in the Law: Draw attention to legislative initiatives that try to improve the assistance that students with dyslexia get in school systems. Talk about how laws and policies tailored to the needs of people with dyslexia affect inclusion.

2. Dyslexia Awareness efforts: Examine how local and international efforts for dyslexia awareness might lessen stigma, promote understanding, and advance an inclusive society.

Individual Development and Self-Empowerment

1. Methods Centered on Strengths: Stress the value of strengths-based learning strategies for both personal growth and education. Honor the special skills and qualities that people with dyslexia contribute to a variety of areas.

2. Self-Advocacy and Mentoring: Talk about the increasing focus on mentoring programs and self-advocacy abilities for dyslexic people. Examine how mentoring relationships may spur professional and personal development.

Constructing a Helpful Ecosystem

1. Partnerships Between Education and Business: Investigate collaborations between academic institutions and business sectors to establish job, internship, and mentoring programs for dyslexics.

2. Community-Based Support Initiatives: Draw attention to neighborhood-based programs that aim to create networks of support for dyslexic people and their families. Talk about the role that neighborhood associations have in fostering a feeling of community.

A Prospective Perspective

As this chapter comes to an end, picture a day when dyslexia is accepted as a vital component of neurodiversity and is not simply understood. Imagine a society in which people with dyslexia are enabled to realize their full potential and where a variety of views are heard.

1. Inclusive Education Practices: Picture a world in which inclusive education techniques are the standard, guaranteeing that all students—dyslexic learners included—get the assistance and modifications they need to succeed.

2. Global Collaboration: Envision a future in which academics, educators, activists, and legislators work together globally to develop novel approaches and exchange best practices for supporting dyslexia.

Final Thoughts
In "Beyond the Letters," consider how we have all come to understand and accept dyslexia in the book's last chapters. Stress the need for ongoing support, advocacy, and education to build a society in which people with dyslexia not only flourish but also take the lead in determining a better future for all.